DOES ATTITUDE OF

PHYSIOTHERAPIST

TOWARDS TREATMENT MATTER?

Nitesh Bansal

ABSTRACT

A Low back pain is reportedly one of the most common musculoskeletal problems that is managed by physiotherapists globally and it constitutes a significant health problem with a heavy economic burden to the patient as well as the community. Physiotherapists treat a large number of patients with low back pain, accounting for approximately half their workload. Studies show that prevalence of LBP among Indian populations ranges from 6.2% to 92%.

Evidence-based treatment for low back pain other than conventional physiotherapy (PT) treatments includes counselling, educational informative sessions, painkillers and exercises under supervision. Guidelines for the treatment of low back pain recommend that practitioners identify risk factors and intervene early.

In managing low back pain, it has been suggested that clinicians focus on factors beyond conventional treatment principles. Importantly, it has been observed that the attitudes and beliefs of the practitioner or clinician significantly impacts the management of a condition/disorder, and consequently the related outcomes. In recent study, it was reported that almost 10% of musculoskeletal physiotherapists will persist in their treatment in non-responsive patients as they believe that their patients will improve, at some point, as there is a cumulative effect. Interestingly, this persistence depends upon the belief of the clinician, and not on available evidence. Accordingly, it is important that factors related to attitudes and beliefs of Indian physiotherapists towards the management of LBP should be comprehensively investigated.

Physiotherapists with at minimum one year of work experience, after completing their base professional degree were identified, and administered a questionnaire that also included the ABS – mp measurement tool. An online version of the survey instrument (s) was created on Survey Monkey, an online solution for conducting surveys. Next the survey was sent electronically to physiotherapists across country. In addition, hard copies were also completed by physiotherapists at conferences and workshops. The data was compiled in Microsoft excel and subsequently analysed using SPSS version 16.

309 valid responses were received from across four zones of the country. The total attitude and belief total score of the Indian physiotherapists sampled was relatively high (95.12 ±12.12), while the means for the sub-domain, personal interaction was 63 (±8.4) and treatment orientation was 31.7 ($\pm$ 5.06). There results suggest the attitudes and beliefs of Indian physiotherapists were dependent on their gender, their qualifications and patient care setups that they worked in across all the domains.

Physiotherapists involved in the management of LBP, regardless of their specialization, scored moderately high on the ABS-mp scale. Taken together, the results suggest that Indian physiotherapists are willing to employ a psychological approach, have a preference to continue therapy for longer periods of time, and are open to referring patients to other experts for opinion. Furthermore and interestingly, it appears that physiotherapists, who primarily use a bio-medical approach, promote a fear of avoidance of movement and/or activity by advising their patients to delay their return to work and limit their physical activity.

Key words: Attitude, Belief, Low Back Pain, Indian Physiotherapists

CONTENTS

LIST OF TABLES

LIST OF FIGURES

LIST OF ABBERIVENTIONS

ABS-mp	Attitude and Back Pain Scale for Musculoskeletal Practitioner
BM	Biomedical
CC	Confidence & Concern
CHS	Connection to Health Care System
IPD	In Patient Department
LBP	Low Back Pain
LS	Limitation on Session
OPD	Out Patient Department
PI	Personal Interaction
PS	Psychological Approach
PT	Physiotherapy
RA	Re-Activation
SD	Standard Deviation
SPSS	Statistical Package for Social Studies
TO	Treatment Orientation
WCPT	World Confederation of Physiotherapy

CHAPTER ONE: INTRODUCTION

1.1 BACKGROUND

Pain is widespread and universal, yet it is not very well understood. Often the best hope for a patient suffering from persistent pain is that it can be adequately managed, assuming it has been identified as a problem by the clinician in the first place. This should be a joint venture between patient and attending physiotherapists and/or other pain clinicians to ensure that the patient's quality of life can be maintained if not improved wherever possible.

Low Back Pain (LBP) continues to present as a significant and challenging health problem around the globe, but especially in developing countries like India. Studies report the prevalence among an Indian population to range from 6.2% to 92%. Furthermore, it constitutes a problem with a heavy economic burden to the patient as well as the community. Physiotherapists are on the fore front in addressing this challenge as Low back pain is the most common musculoskeletal condition seen by physical therapists in developed countries. (Philadelphia panel 2001, Australian Acute Musculoskeletal Pain Guidelines Group 2003).

Low back pain is a descriptive term that manifests as a result of injury to muscles, ligaments, intervertebral discs and other connective tissues located in the low back area. Reasons for injury can be aberrant loading and stress on tissues due to inactivity due to modern life styles, manual handling, repetitive movements and/or sustained incorrect postures (Morris C 2006). Psychological constructs such as, pre-existing depression, anxiety, fear avoidance behaviour, poor coping strategies, and social factors, like workplace environment can also negatively impact low back pain. It is suggested that psychosocial factors can contribute significantly, from mild to moderate disability or sometimes even severe disability and distress in patients suffering from LBP (Walker BF 2000). It is now well established that chronicity of Low back pain and its disability is not comprehensively explained exclusively by physical or biological factors, but are also influenced to a large extent by psychosocial constructs. Thus, its management should include not only treating physical/ biological parameters but also psychological and social constructs. (Stanley Innes 2015)

The approach towards treatment of low back pain is rapidly changing from only biomedical approach to bio-psychological approach. Attitudes and beliefs about the treatment of low back pain through biopsychosocial model, its course and management plays an important role as they impact on the low back pain individuals comprehensively. This further impacts severity and extent of disability and distress causes by the condition. The clinical guidelines recommend evaluation of bio-psychological factors when deciding on patient's management.

Evidence based treatment for non-specific low back pain not only include conventional physiotherapy management but also brief educational interventions, Pain relieving medications, graded and supervised exercise and counselling (Ladeira CE, 2011). Clinical practice guidelines recommend evaluation of bio-psychological factors when deciding on patient's management. Though several systematic reviews have identified several risk factors for the development of persistent pain, the contribution of each of the risk factors to pain is considerably small. (Pincus T et al. 2002) Furthermore, almost all guidelines recommend early intervention and urge practitioners to identify and consider risk factors in pain management, but offer little specific guidance as to how they might address these risk factors during their clinical practice. Hence, the implementation of these guidelines has proved difficult and, where implemented, they have made little impact on practice. (Little P et al., 1996 and Barnett AG, Underwood MR, Vickers MR 1999)

Several studies have argued that rather than focusing exclusively on risk factors and differences in patient symptoms and their management, factors attributable to the clinician need to be investigated (Pincus T et al., 2002; Foster NE et al., 2003). It has been observed that practitioner's attitudes and beliefs, leads to over treating or under treating the low back pain, failing to refer appropriately, and over time reinforcing illness perception through advice for complete bed rest, to be extra careful while carrying out normal activities of daily living, reducing their activity levels etc. Accordingly, this further reinforces the pain behaviour of LBP patients. (Bishop A, Foster NE. 2005, Darlow et al 2012). This eventually take the low back pain to chronicity level and subsequently to long term disability. Interestingly, there is good evidence that some clinicians advise mobility while others believe that painful movements should be avoided – leading to fear avoidance rather than protected mobility (Linton SJ, Vlaeyen J, Ostelo RJ. 2002). Thus, attitudes and beliefs of health care professionals has an impact not only on his / her clinical decision making, but also on the attitude and belief of patients towards their particular condition. It acts like two-way sword.

 In summary, clinical guidelines exist for the management of back pain, but they are not comprehensively followed. This is reflected by the varied advice given by physiotherapists and their choice of treatment, which interestingly are not consistent with the guidelines in most cases. Attitudes and beliefs can significantly contribute to the development of low back pain (LBP) and disability in a number of ways, including the degree and intensity of treatment, the lack of or overuse of effective pain control or reactivation strategies, reinforcing patient's unhelpful illness perceptions by advising increased spinal care, and restricting or limiting normal activities. *Pincus T et al.. (2006)* reported that over 10% (lower estimate) of all musculoskeletal physiotherapy practitioners continue to treat patients with sub-acute back pain, even if they are not responding as well as expected. Furthermore, and more importantly clinicians continue to disregard guidelines for the treatment of low back pain that have been formulated based on evidence.

1.2 NEED OF THE STUDY

Worldwide, Low back pain is one of the most prevalent musculoskeletal condition treated by physiotherapists. There are well established guidelines that outline the conventional management of low back pain. However, it is also true that the attitudes and beliefs of physiotherapists play an important role in the management of patients with LBP. Furthermore, it is purported that these attitudes and beliefs are significantly impacted by the diversity of India with regards to its population, and cultural belief system. Thus, it is important to study the attitudes and beliefs of Indian Physiotherapists managing LBP.

A study of a clinician's attitudes and beliefs with regards to the management of LBP, will help highlight the importance of attitudinal and belief systems in the management of LBP and also modify current conventional treatment guidelines. The uniformity and standardization of LBP treatment is important in the effective rehabilitation of patients with this disabling condition and consequently help facilitate the return to work and improve their quality of life. A novel understanding of this dimension in managing LBP will assist policy makers, and other professionals involved create universal policies to effectively manage patients with LBP across clinical setups and geographies.

1.3 AIMS, REASEARCH QUESTIONS & OBJECTIVES

AIMS:

The aim of this study was to investigate the attitudes and beliefs of Indian physiotherapists towards the management of back pain. Secondly, to study the association between attitudes and beliefs and education, gender, geography, use of guidelines, types of patient care setups, therapist specialization, and types of interventions etc.

RESEARCH QUESTIONS:

1. What are the attitudes and beliefs of Indian physiotherapists in managing of LBP?

2. Is there an association between attitudes and beliefs with the treating Physiotherapists education, their gender, the geography they worked in, their use of guidelines, the types of patient care setups they worked in, the therapist specialization, and the types of interventions that they used?

OBJECTIVES:

1. To determine attitudes and beliefs of Indian physiotherapists towards the management of Low Back Pain

2. To compare the attitudes and beliefs of Indian physiotherapists towards the management of Low Back Pain across different geographical zones.

3. To compare the attitudes and beliefs of Indian physiotherapists towards the management of Low Back Pain across gender.

4. To compare the attitudes and beliefs of Indian physiotherapists towards the management of Low Back Pain as a function of educational qualifications.

5. To compare the attitudes and beliefs of Indian physiotherapists towards the management of Low Back Pain across therapist specializations.

6. To compare the attitudes and beliefs of Indian physiotherapists towards the management of Low Back Pain as a function of type of interventions.

7.   To compare the attitudes and beliefs of Indian physiotherapists towards the management of Low Back Pain across different patient care Set ups.

8.   To compare the attitudes and beliefs of Indian physiotherapists towards the management of Low Back Pain with the use of guidelines.

1.4 HYPOTHESES

$H_0$1:

There is no significant difference in attitude & belief of Indian Physiotherapists towards management of low back pain across different geographical zones.

H_a1:

There is a significant difference in attitude & belief of Indian Physiotherapists towards management of low back pain across different geographical zones.

$H_0$2:

There is no significant difference in attitude & belief of Indian Physiotherapists towards management of low back pain across different genders.

H_a2:

There is a significant difference in attitude & belief of Indian Physiotherapists towards management of low back pain across different genders.

$H_0$3:

There is no significant difference in attitude & belief of Indian Physiotherapists towards management of low back pain across different educational qualifications.

H_a3:

There is a significant difference in attitude & belief of Indian Physiotherapists towards management of low back pain across different educational qualifications.

$H_0$4:

There is no significant difference in attitude & belief of Indian Physiotherapists towards management of low back pain across different therapist specializations.

H_a4:

There is a significant difference in attitude & belief of Indian Physiotherapists towards management of low back pain across different therapist specializations.

H$_0$5:

There is no significant difference in attitude & belief of Indian Physiotherapists towards management of low back pain across different types of Interventions.

H$_a$5:

There is a significant difference in attitude & belief of Indian Physiotherapists towards management of low back pain across different types of Interventions.

H$_0$6:

There is no significant difference in attitude & belief of Indian Physiotherapists towards management of low back pain across different patient care set-ups.

H$_a$6:

There is a significant difference in attitude & belief of Indian Physiotherapists towards management of low back pain across different patient care set-ups.

H$_0$7:

There is no significant difference in attitude & belief of Indian Physiotherapists towards management of low back pain with the use of guidelines.

H$_a$7:

There is a significant difference in attitude & belief of Indian Physiotherapists towards management of low back pain with the use of guidelines.

CHAPTER TWO: REVIEW OF LITERATURE

2.1 LOW BACK PAIN:

2.1.1 PREVALENCE

Low back pain is a major health problem and is third most commonly reported symptom. It is defined as pain, muscle tension or stiffness located below the costal margins and above the inferior gluteal folds, with or without leg pain. The cause or the triggering stimulus of pain maybe as a result of damage to either muscle, fascia, bone, ligament, intervertebral disc, and/or nerve (Balagué, F et al. 2012). Interestingly, a majority of the LBP cases may have multiple causes and sometimes do not have clear cause (Casazza BA, 2012).

A systemic review by Walker BF, et al. (2000) reported that the point prevalence of low back pain ranges from 12%- 33%, however the lifetime prevalence ranges from 11%- 84%. Others have reported a lifetime prevalence of 50-80% (Cohen et al., 2008); and 6.2% to 92% (Bindra et al., 2015). It has been reported that LBP is more prevalent in females and adults in the age group of 40-80 years (Chou, R., Qaseem, A., et al. 2007), while others have observed it afflicting males and females in equal numbers (National institute of neurological disorders, 2016). In studying nature and occurrence pattern of LBP, Croft et al. (1998) found that low back pain is the condition that relapses in more than 75% of the cases and only some patients recover completely within 12 months after the first consultation.

2.1.2 MORBIDITY

Low back pain is a major cause of morbidity globally, as it affects a person not only biologically, but also socioeconomically and psychologically. According to Melloh M et al. (2008), LBP is responsible for high treatment costs, increased sick leave, individual suffering, and is one of the leading causes for people to seek health care services. Yet surprisingly, to date it has been relatively under-prioritised and under-funded. Hoy D et al. (2010) have proposed that one important reason for this may be the low ranking LBP received relative to other conditions in the Global Burden of Disease rankings. However, it has been gaining attention, and is now one of the most frequent conditions reported by patients seeking medical care (Woodwell DA 1995).

2.1.3 CLASSIFICATION AND ETIOLOGY

The lower back consists of 5 lumbar vertebrae, the sacrum and the coccyx, which are functionally interconnected and supported by a number of muscles, ligaments, fascia, intervertebral disc, spinal cord and nerve roots. Figure 2.1 represents the anatomy of Low back.

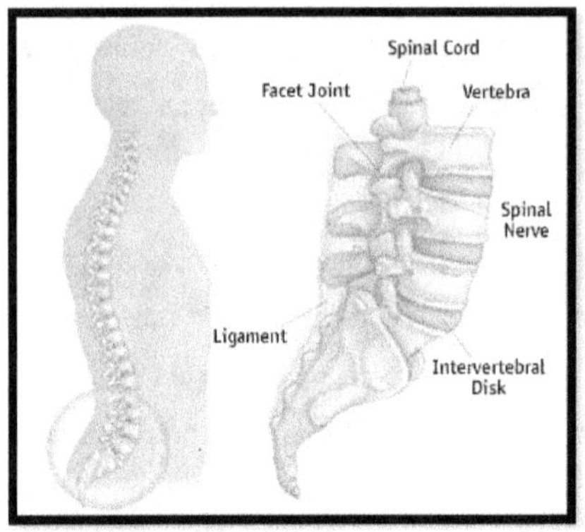

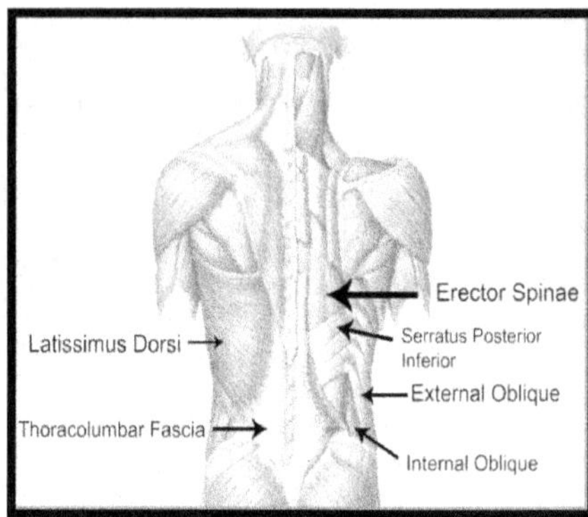

Image source: orthoinfo.aaos.

Image Source: http://canacopegdl.com

Figure 2.1: Diagrammatic representation of anatomy of low back region, muscles.

Low back pain can be triggered or arise from dysfunction of any one or all of these structure. Most often low back pain is classified on the basis of duration as acute, sub-acute and chronic low back pain, and plays a vital role in assessing the prognosis of the condition. It is observed that more than 5 to 10% of acute and subacute low back pain cases become chronic, which the has a significant impact on the patient's quality of life, and additionally disability as a result of chronic LBP has been strongly associated with psychosocial dysfunction (Gunnar BJ and Andersson MD, 1999).

Others, such as Mackenzie 1981, have classified low back pain on the basis of underlying causative factors, as mechanical, non-mechanical or chemical. Mechanical pain comes from deformation of structures containing nociceptive nerve endings. In this type of LBP there is a strong association between patient symptoms and body postures, with changing pain levels with positional variations. This includes non-specific musculoskeletal strains, herniated discs, compressed nerve roots, degenerative discs or joint disease, and broken vertebra. In contrast, non- mechanical or chemical types of LBP are constant in nature, and it is possible that certain body positions may increase pain, however no positional adjustments will relives the pain. This includes tumors, inflammatory conditions such as spondylitis, and infections. Thus, the causes and consequences of LBP are multifactorial. (Refer Figure 2.2)

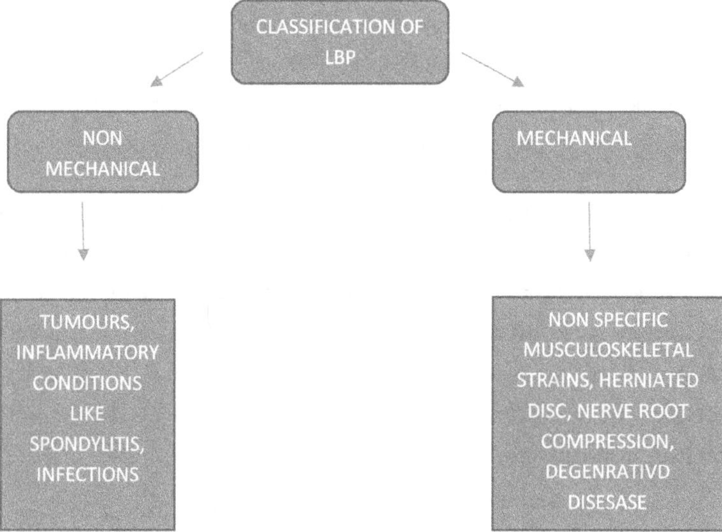

Figure 2.2: Schematic representation of Classification of Low Back Pain

2.1.4 BIOPSYCHOLOGICAL MODEL

The biopsychosocial model was proposed by George L. Engel in 1977 to reflect the development of illness through the complex interaction of biological factors, psychological factors and social factors. The biological factors mainly includes genetic, biochemical etc. Psychological factors like mood, personality, behaviour, etc. and social factors like cultural, familial, socioeconomic, medical, etc. This model was proposed to find an alternate to biomedical model which has been a dominant health care model since many years. According to Wade and Halligan 2017, biomedical model is still as dominant in health care system.

The 'bio' component of this theory examines aspects of biology that influence health. These might include things like brain changes, genetics, or functioning of major body organs, such as the liver, the kidneys, or even the motor system. The 'psycho' component of the theory examines psychological components, things like thoughts, emotions, or behaviors. The changes in thoughts due to biological mal functioning might lead to changes in behaviors, like avoiding certain situations, staying at home, or quitting job. As person engages in these behaviors, injury might worsen, or could suffer further depression and anxiety. The 'social' component of the BPS model examines social factors that might influence the health of an individual, things like our interactions with others, our culture, or our economic status. Being unable to fulfill the social role might trigger problems and increase the stress that could lead to further biological or psychological problems.

The national institute of health and clinical excellence 2009, emphasized on the use of bio-psychological model for the management of low back pain. The biopsychosocial model acknowledges the patient as a whole, their social, cultural and environmental aspects influences an individual's response to illness. Thus we can say it is a patient-centric healthcare system. According to Liddle, Baxter and Gracey 2007, physiotherapy has begun to embrace the biopsychosocial model. But there is question about how to utilize it effectively in management of back pain.

As seen in Figure 2.3, the risk factors for the low back pain can be categorised into sociodemographic, behavioural, biological, psychological and psychosocial factors. Where Biological factors emphasis on biological process or physical malfunctioning of the body. Further, psychological and social factors emphasis on attitude, belief, perception etc. and interpersonal relationships respectively.

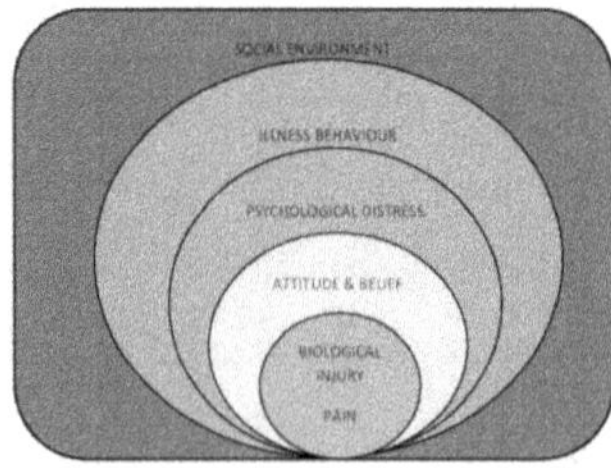

Figure 2.3: Biopsychological model of back pain

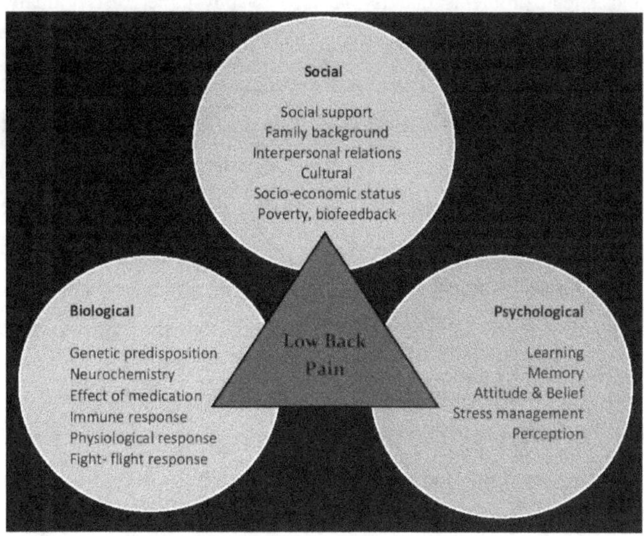

Figure.2.4: Schematic presentation of description of bio-psychological model for pain.

The traditional management of Low Back Pain has focused primarily on a biomedical approach, which is dependent on a biomedical model of the disease. Thus, treatment approaches based on this model focus entirely on the biological/physical pathology and accordingly address physical symptoms and impairments (Daykin AR and Richardson B 2004; Foster NE 2005). However, as shown in Fig.2.4, there is definite influence of various components i.e. biological, psychological and social factors on the health and condition of a person. Thus, for the comprehensive rehabilitation of a person suffering from Low back pain a clinician needs base his/her management on the tripartite biopsychosocial model and consider all factors that contribute to LBP.

2.1.4 INTERVENTIONS

There are a wide variety of treatment approaches available for low back pain. Generally, the management of low back pain (LBP) involves a multifaceted approach with a primary objective relieving a patient's pain, and consequently restoring discomfort free function. The management of LBP ranges from life style modification, medicines, physiotherapy, yoga, osteopathy, acupuncture, psychological counselling to surgical procedures.

Maniadakis & Gray (2000) reported that Low back pain (LBP) is one of the most common musculoskeletal problems that is managed by physiotherapists globally. Physiotherapy interventions include exercise, manual therapy, heat/cold, electrical modalities etc. Foster et al. (2015) have suggested the treatment plans that stratified care were an appropriate approach. Stratified care is the targeting of treatment to subgroups of patients based on musculoskeletal characteristics and parameters. Accordingly, there are three (3) different approaches to stratification that have shown beneficial results: prognosis of patient, responsiveness of treatment and underlying mechanism. However, the use of these different stratification strategies vary around the world and there are also several degrees of overlap between these three different approaches (Foster et al. 2015).

A systemic review by Ledeira 2011, reported that after patient education, spine mobilization/ manipulation and exercise i.e. stabilization and directional preference were the most common therapeutic intervention recommended for patients with non-specific acute LBP. Castro Sanchez et al. 2016, reported that In comparison to functional technique, spinal manipulative therapy showed greater reduction in disability in patients with chronic LBP. Dougherty et al. (2014) also reported that spinal manipulation techniques are effective in reducing pain and disability in Low back pain when compared to sham group. According to a systemic review by Luca MChiro et al. 2017, there are limited evidences which have studied the effectiveness of spinal manipulations. Nagrale et al. 2012, supported the use of spinal mobilization along with spinal stabilization exercises for treating non radicular low back pain.

Karthikeyan, Moorthy and Pradnya 2015 studied efficacy of Mulligan technique for the management of Low Back Pain. The study reported that the mulligan technique is effective in management of non-radicular LBP. Further, lumbar spine mobilization and exercise was beneficial in reducing short-term disability and improving pain.

There are various schools of thought exist for spinal mobilization. Namely, Maitland, mulligan are widely used by Physiotherapists. According to Maitland, Hengeveld, Banks, and English, 2005, a Passive accessory intervertebral movement (PAIVM) is a mobilisation technique that produces movement of a mobile vertebral segment without active participation of muscles related to the movement.

Movement with mobilization is a manual therapy technique which was developed by Brian Mulligan, for the treatment of musculoskeletal dysfunction. It involves performing a sustained force (accessory glide) while a previously painful (problematic) movement is performed. Jonas. (2005) and Vicenzino. (2009).

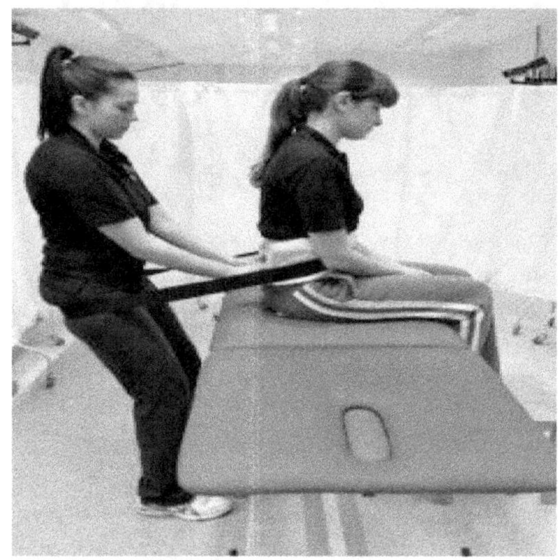

Image Source: www.physio-pedia.com/

Figure 2.5: Movement with mobilization (MWM) technique for Low back Pain

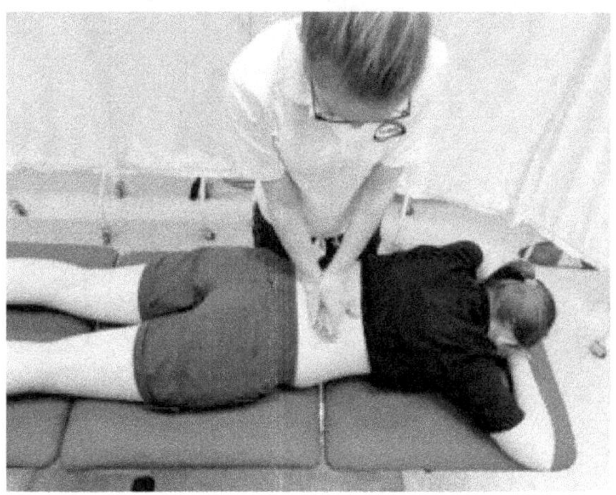

Image Source: www.physio-pedia.com/

Figure 2.6: Central Postero-anterior (PA) mobilization technique

Spinal muscle stretching, strengthening exercises, Core stabilization exercises play an important role in low back pain management.

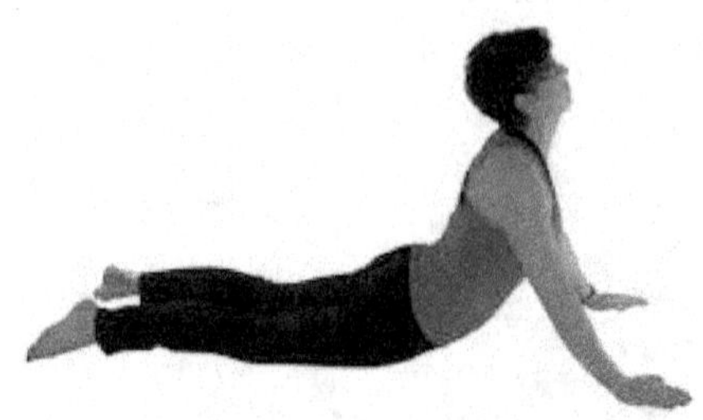

Image Source: http://www.stretching-exercises-guide.com

Figure 2.7: Example of stretching exercises

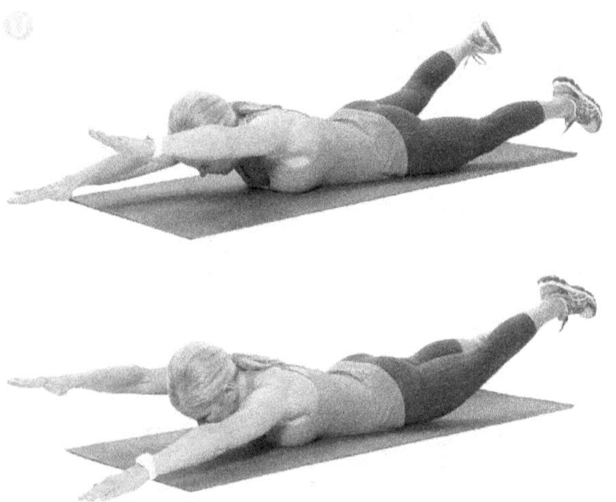

Image source: https://gethealthyu.com/exercise/mid-back-extension

Figure 2.8: Example of strengthening exercises

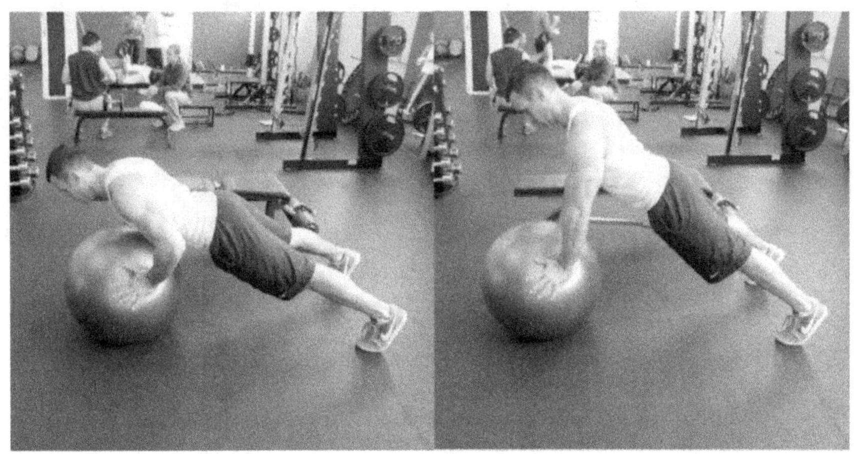

Figure 2.9: Example of Core stabilization exercises

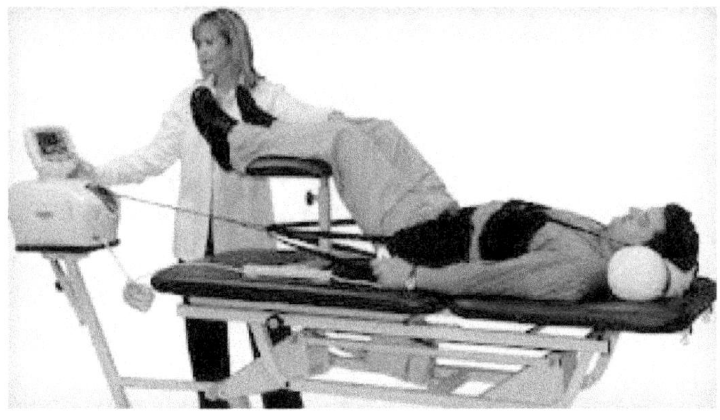

Image source: sportsperformanceandspine.com

Figure 2.10: Spinal Traction Unit (Lumbar region)

A wide variety of therapeutic interventions are used around the world, but by far the most utilized are a variety of manual therapy techniques that are based on diverse theoretical constructs (Foster, et al. 1999). Furthermore, and in addition the most commonly used electrotherapeutic modalities are interferential therapy, ultrasound, pulsed short-wave diathermy, and transcutaneous electrical nerve stimulation and Traction.

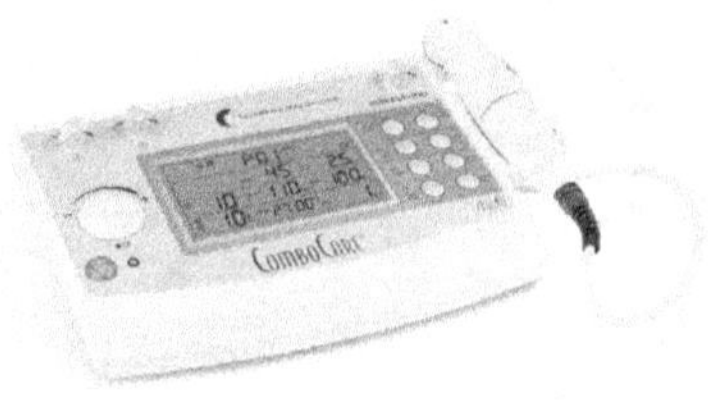

Image Source: www.tensunits.com

Figure 2.11: Ultrasound and TENS

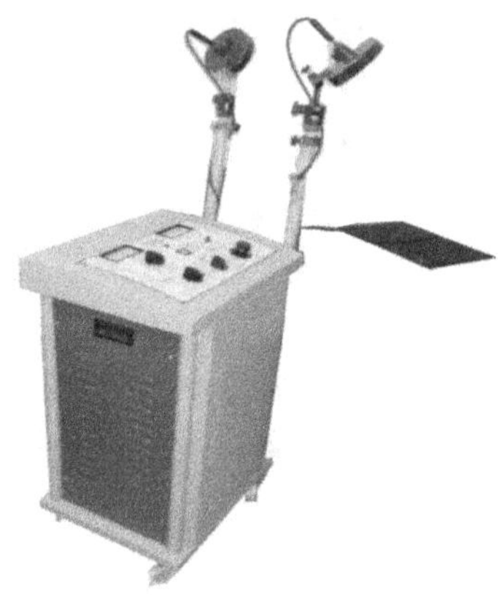

Image source: www.doctortechindia.com

Figure 2.12: Short wave diathermy

More recently, it has been reported that in keeping with current guidelines and evidence based practice, low back pain is treated principally using some specific types of manual techniques and educational advice (Gracey J et al., 2002). Praneet and colleagues found that hospital based physiotherapists used electrotherapeutic modalities to larger extent than university linked clinicians, who used more manual therapy techniques. This suggests that university based physiotherapists integrate current guidelines to a greater extent than hospital based therapists, as current research based evidence has reported an advantage of benefits in the management of LBP with manual therapy techniques over electrotherapy modalities. (Praneet et al., 2004).

2.2 ATITUDES AND BELIEFS IN THE MANAGEMENT OF LBP

A belief is an idea that a person holds as being true. A person can base a belief upon certainties (e.g. mathematical principles), probabilities or matters of faith. Belief of an individual come from either a person's own experiences or experiments or the acceptance of cultural and societal norms (e.g. religion) or what other people say (e.g. education or mentoring). On the other hand, attitudes are the mental dispositions people have towards others and the current circumstances before making decisions that result in behavior. People primarily form their attitudes from underlying values and beliefs. But the factors which may not have been internalized as beliefs and values can still influence a person's attitudes at the point of decision-making. Typical influences include the desire to please, political correctness, convenience, peer pressure, and psychological stressors. According to Alport 1954, Ketz and Stotland 1959, the belief is cognitive aspect and attitude is affective or motivational aspect.

The concept of attitude – behavior relations, is fairly old, but its use in the management of pain is relatively new and is progressively gaining acceptance worldwide. It has been argued that an assessment of attitudes should be included as part of a multidimensional assessment prior to the commencement of treatment programmes *(Strong et al. 1990)*.

Guidelines pertaining to the management of Low back pain have been in existence for many years, but the adherence to these by health care professionals remains scarce (Bishop et al., 2003). The reason for this non adherence may lie in the attitude and belief of the health care professionals as they are dependent on a diverse number of factors. Rainville J et al. (1995) did a study to find out the attitudes and beliefs of Health care providers about functional impairments and chronic back pain and concluded that clinicians have been shown to hold a range of beliefs and attitudes about pain. Daykin & Richardson (2004) and Vlaeyen & Linton (2006) observed that attitudes and beliefs of a practitioner impacts management and consequently outcomes. These include over or under treating, referrals to appropriate specialists when patients do not respond to treatment etc. The therapist's attitudes and beliefs, contribute to the development of chronic spinal disability by over treating or under treating, failing to refer appropriately, and, in time, reinforcing illness perception through advice to increase spinal and environmental vigilance while restricting normal activities. Thus it is extremely important to know the attitude and belief of physiotherapists regarding management of low back pain.

In his work, Houben et al. (2004) suggested that practitioner's attitudes and beliefs were consistently associated with recommendations for work and physical activity for patients (based on clinical vignettes). Hence, there is some support that practitioners' beliefs and attitudes influence their behaviour (such as the information they provide to patients)

Several measurement scales have been developed to measure attitudes and beliefs of clinicians towards the management of pain. For an example, the Pain Attitudes and Beliefs Scale for Physiotherapists (PABT.PT) by Ostelo et al. (2003), the Health Care Providers' Pain and Impairment Relationship Scale developed by Rainville et al. (1995), Backs beliefs questionnaire, the physical sub-section of the Fear-avoidance belief questionnaire Linton et al. (2002) etc.

The Pain and Impairment Relationship Scale (PAIRS) was devised to measure the extent to which patients with chronic pain believe that pain interferes with their functioning (Riley et al. 1988). It consists of 15 items scored on a 7-point Likert scale. A limitation of the PAIRS is its consideration of one attitude alone – that of the pain-impairment link. The Survey of Pain Attitudes (SOPA) instrument consists of 24 true false items arranged into 5 subscales: medical cure, pain control, solicitude, disability and medication *(Jensen et al. 1987)*. The revised instrument of SOPA *(Jensen & Karoly 1987)* contains the 5 subscales of the earlier version plus a 6th subscale which taps the attitude that pain may be influenced by an emotional link.

More recently, Pincus T et al. (2006) in order to evaluate practitioner's beliefs and attitudes to the treatment of low back pain, and whether these influence their clinical decisions, intervention strategies, and patient-centred outcomes; developed and tested a new questionnaire, the Attitudes to Back Pain Scale (ABS), for a specific group of clinicians, practitioners who specialize in musculoskeletal therapy. Pincus (2006) also reported that this tool was valid and reliable instrument. Similarly, Bishop et al. (2007) reported that a factor analysis of the Abs-mp had established validity, but reliability was not explicitly tested.

Foster et al (2003) argued that clinician factors need investigating to better understand the complexity of professional practice behaviour and how to improve implementation of guidelines in LBP management. Kennedy N. et al (2014) compared beliefs of students of medicine, physiotherapy and nursing (total of 271) towards low back pain. They concluded that differences exist in the beliefs of three cohorts of students toward LBP.

Pincus T et al. (2007) investigated the attitudes of three professional groups, namely Chiropractors, Osteopaths and Physiotherapists, who play key roles in the management of low back pain (LBP) patients using a recently developed and validated questionnaire, the Attitudes to Back Pain Scale for musculoskeletal practitioners (ABS-mp). A survey was sent to 300 of each professional group of (n=900). After analysing the responses, they concluded that all three groups endorse a psychosocial approach to treatment, and see re-activation as a primary goal. However, physiotherapists and osteopaths tend to endorse attitudes towards limiting the number of treatment sessions offered to LBP patients more than chiropractors, and chiropractors endorse a more biomedical approach than physiotherapists.

Clinicians have been shown to hold a range of beliefs and attitudes about pain, and these appear to be related to the recommendations and treatment they give to patients. Previous research has suggested that the uptake of guidelines by professional groups is related to practitioner's beliefs and attitudes. Yet very little literature exists on evaluation of attitudes amongst Indian Physiotherapists working in different settings, towards low back pain.

A systematic review reported moderate evidence regarding the presence of fear avoidance beliefs amongst practitioners. This, it was suggested leads to unnecessary prescriptions for leave, rest and reduce activity by practitioners. It further reinforces pain behaviour of the patients, consequently leading to more disability (Darlow B, 2012). Thus, it was purported that attitudes and beliefs of a practitioner has a significant impact on the treatment approach used and also on the patient's attitude and belief related to the condition and their own health. There are a fair number of studies that have been related to attitudes and beliefs of general physician, chiropractitioners, and nursing related to treatment interventions and health (Gardener T et al 2017), however, there is a paucity of literature that relates to evaluating attitudes and beliefs of Indian Physiotherapists working with patients suffering from low back pain.

2.3 RESEARCH GAPS

According to the literature, Low back pain is major health problem faced worldwide. The management of low back pain needs to be multi- dimensional, with a focus not merely on the biological domain, but also the psychological and social domains (Biopsychosocial model). Physiotherapy as a profession has taken steps to integrate this model within its clinical practice, however several gaps in its theoretical knowledge and its practical approach in the management of LBP. Various physiotherapy treatment options are available to treat low back pain and several studies have been conducted in recent years to evaluate the effectiveness of manual therapy, electrotherapy and exercise protocols for managing low back pain (Foster, et al. 1999, Gracey J et al., 2002, Praneet et al. 2004). Guidelines for managing LBP have been available for some time, but adherence to them are a problem. It is possible that a major hurdle to their implementation is the attitudes and beliefs of the clinician. Several researchers (Daykin & Richardson, 2004,; Vlaeyen & Linton, 2006) have suggested that the attitudes and beliefs of a practitioner plays an important role in deciding the management of a condition, and consequently the choice of intervention and its outcome. Several studies have evaluated the attitudes and beliefs of clinicians in a diverse group of health care professionals. However, very few studies have been done on physiotherapists who managing low back pain (e.g., Pincus T et al. 2007). In contrast to Western societies, the Indian health environment is divergently different, in terms of not only geography but also ethnicity, culture, etc., and thus, attitudes and beliefs. Accordingly, studies that evaluate attitudes and beliefs of Indian physiotherapists in delivering health interventions need to be conducted to develop comprehensive models of healthcare services.

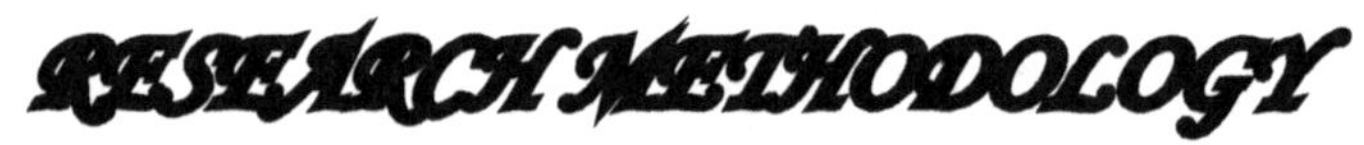
RESEARCH METHODOLOGY

CHAPTER THREE: RESEARCH METHODOLOGY

This chapter deals with research methodology used for the study which includes participants, study design, sampling techniques and procedure.

3.1 PARTICIPANTS:

The study was conducted on qualified and practicing Indian Physiotherapists across four zones (North, South, East and West) of India. The following inclusion and exclusion criteria was used:

3.1.1 INCLUSION CRITERIA:

As a physiotherapist an individual can work in various set ups ranging from clinical setup to hospital set up to academic institutions. The work environment is different in each set ups. The attitude and belief can be influenced by policies of the set up. Thus it is important to include therapists from various working set ups. Further, physiotherapists also work as specialists in particular condition or area of health care like Physiotherapy in neurological conditions, Sports, Musculoskeletal conditions, gynaecological conditions. Thus it is important to target the physiotherapists who work with the Low back pain patients. Keeping all these aspects in mind the Physiotherapists who met the following criteria were included in the study:

- Physiotherapists working in government hospitals, private clinic, private hospitals, academic institutes and private practitioners.

- Males and females

- Physiotherapist with at least one year of experience after completing the degree.

- Physiotherapists working with patients with low back pain.

3.1.2 EXCLUSION CRITERIA:

The physiotherapists who are not practising might be not aware about current researches, guidelines for management of low back pain. Further, their attitude and belief may be based on hypothetical situation as they are not involved in every day dealing of the patients with low back pain. Thus the physiotherapists with the following criteria were excluded from the study.

- Non practicing clinical physiotherapists were excluded from the study.

3.2 STUDY DESIGN

The current study aimed to study not only the attitude and belief of Physiotherapists but also compare it across the geographical presentation, working set up, gender, adherence to guidelines etc.

A cross sectional study is a type of observational study that analyses data from a target population, or a representative subset, at a specific point in time, that is cross-sectional data. As the study was conducted on physiotherapists across India at a given time, this study was categorised as a cross sectional study.

Survey study is a method for collecting information or data as reported by individuals. It is an efficient way of gathering data to help answer a research question. Surveys are questionnaires (or a series of questions) that are administered to research participants who answer the questions themselves. Since the participants are providing the information, it is referred to as self-report data. Surveys are used to get an idea of how a group or population feels about a number of things. In the current study, we used the ABS-mp questionnaire to gather information regarding attitudes and beliefs of the Indian Physiotherapists in managing Low back pain. Thus, the study also falls under survey design.

Thus the study design of this study was a Cross sectional, Survey design.

3.3 SAMPLING TECHNIQUE:

Non- probability, convenience sampling.

3.4 SAMPLE SIZE:

Slovins's formula is used to calculate an appropriate sample size from a population. If we do not have any idea about a population's behaviour, we need to use Slovin's formula to find the sample size. The formula was formulated by Slovin in 1961.The sample size for this study was calculated by **Slovin's formula (1961)** which is as follows:

$$n = \frac{N}{1 + Ne^2}$$

Where, n= Sample size

N= Population (Approximate target population size, N= 50000)

e= margin error (e= 0.5)

n= 50000/ 1+ 50000 * $(0.05)^2$

n= 50000/ 1+ 50000* 0.0025

n= 50000/ 1+ 125

n= 396.82= 397

Considering the attrition, we have to adjust the sample size by following formula (**KP Suresh, S. Chandrashekhara 2012**):

N_1= N/ 1-q

Where, N_1= adjusted sample size

N= calculated sample size (397)

q= proportion of attrition which is considered as 10% for our study.

N_1= 397/1- 0.1

N_1= 397/ 0.9

N_1= 441

Sample size= 441

3.5 INSTRUMENT:

A self-administered questionnaire with two parts was used to achieve the aims and objectives of the study. (Appendix II)

Part A: Included the demographic and professional details of physiotherapists.

As seen in Appendix II, this section contained questions regarding the age, gender, maximum qualification achieved by the physiotherapist, type of work setting, number of patients seen per day. This part also included questions regarding how much time the therapist dedicated towards clinical care and administrative work during the duty hours.

Part B: Included the ABS – mp questionnaire.

The ABS-mp questionnaire consists of two sections: Personal Interaction (PI) and Treatment Orientation (TO). A total of 19 questions are included, which are scored on 7-point Likert scale that ranges from extremely disagree to extremely agree.

Personal interaction (PI) section has thirteen (13) questions, of which five (5) questions are reverse scored. PI is further divided into the following four (4) subdomains:

- **Limitations on sessions (LS)**, items about practitioners' policy towards limiting the length of treatment (four items).
- **Psychological (PS)**, items measuring practitioners' willingness to engage with psychological issues with their patients (four items).
- **Connection to healthcare system (CHS)**, items measuring practitioners' perception of the health-care system and provision of available services (three items).
- **Confidence and concern (CC)**, items measuring practitioners' confidence and concern about treatment and clinical limitations in themselves and others (two items).

Treatment orientation (TO) section includes six (6) questions, and consists of the following two subdomains:

- **Re-activation (RA)**, items that concern return to work and to daily activity and increasing mobility (three items).
- **Biomedical (BM)**; items that concern advice to restrict activities and to be vigilant, and the belief that there is an underlying structural cause of back pain (3 items).

A total score and two sub-scores are calculated by simply adding up individual item scores. The total score ranges from Score of LS and PS domain ranges from 4-28, CHS, RA and BM domain ranges from 3-21 and CC domain ranges from 2-14. The total score of PI section can range between13 to 91 and TO section can range between 6 to 42.

3.5.1 INTERNAL CONSISTENCY OF ABS-MP QUESTIONNAIRE IN INDIAN PHYSIOTHERAPISTS:

Pincus et al. (2006) developed and tested the ABS- mp questionnaire and reported that the questionnaire to be valid and reliable.

Internal consistency or reliability is a measure of item-reliability that establishes if the items addressing the construct being measured are consistent and thus, is dependent on clarity and the derived meaning or understanding of the item. As beliefs, attitudes and clinical practice are influenced by culture, psychological and social dimensions, it is important to establish the internal consistency. Given that India has a widely diverse population – biologically, psychologically, socially and culturally, it was prudent that as a first step, to establish the internal consistency or item-reliability of the ABS – mp in a sample of diverse Indian physiotherapists.

To establish the internal consistency of the survey instrument which consists of a demographic section and the ABS – mp was mailed to 250 Indian physiotherapists around the country using survey monkey, an online survey instrument. Two reminders were given on regular intervals to the physiotherapists to complete the questionnaire. The 147 valid questionnaires were received by March 2017 were compiled in Microsoft excel and analysed by SPSS version 16. Internal Consistency was evaluated by Cronbach alpha coefficient.

The results showed that, the Cronbach alpha coefficient for internal Consistency of ABS-mp was 0. 746. Thus, we can conclude that ABS-mp questionnaire has an adequate internal consistency. Hence this scale can be used for cross sectional study in Indian Physiotherapists (Bansal et al, 2018).

3.6 PROCEDURE:

As a first step, a data base of practicing physiotherapists across India was acquired from professional bodies like the all India Indian Association of Physiotherapists, similar state bodies, conference databases and Society of Indian Physiotherapists etc. Physiotherapist with at minimum one year of work experience after completing their base professional degree were identified and solicited for answering the research survey/questionnaire and the ABS – mp measurement tool. The Online version of the measurement instrument (s) was created with the help of Survey Monkey, an online solution for conducting surveys. The survey was sent electronically to physiotherapists across country. Two reminders were given at regular intervals to the physiotherapists to complete the questionnaire. (Appendix I). Hardcopies were also completed by physiotherapists at conferences and workshops.

Data Reduction and Analysis:

Completed surveys on survey monkey generated the raw data on an excel sheet. While data from the manually filled surveys were entered into the same excel sheet by the primary investigator. Answers were coded and entered to questions that were 'reversed scored' using the tool available in Microsoft excel.

The data thus compiled in Microsoft excel* was subsequently analysed using SPSS** version 16. Descriptive statistics, central tendencies were reported. After initial descriptive analysis, we found that the number of participants under 'educational qualifications', work settings' and the 'interventions used' categories were small and the data were skewed. Thus, data across groups were collapsed under two groups i.e. undergraduate and post graduate for further comparative analysis. Similarly, the data across groups of interventions used by Physiotherapists and work setting were also collapsed. Intervention groups were collapsed under manual therapy and others, and Electrotherapy plus both. The work settings groups were collapsed under out-patient department and in-patient department plus both. Further, appropriate non-parametric tests were used to make comparisons between groups where needed. Non parametric tests were used as the measurement tool used was based on an ordinal scale, the groups had unequal sample sizes, and the data did not meet the assumptions of normality. The Mann Whitney 'U' was used for two independent groups and the Kruskal wallis 'χ^2' for comparisons across more than two groups. A p<0.05 was used where required to test for significance. (Refer Fig.3.1)

*Microsoft excel Version 2013   **SPSS Statistics software: IBM, version 16.0

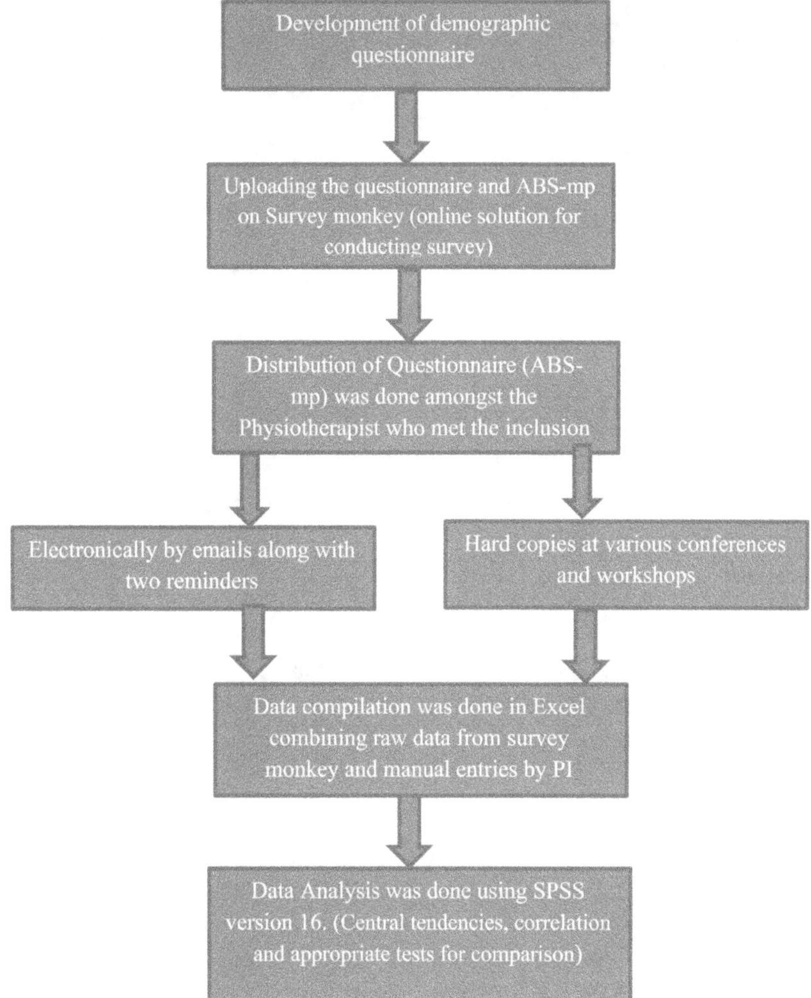

Figure 3.1: Schematic presentation of Procedure followed for the research.

RESULTS

CHAPTER FOUR: RESULTS

4.1 DEMOGRAPHICS

Of the 441 self-administered questionnaire, there were 309 valid responses, which were further analysed. One hundred and thirty two (132) surveys were deemed invalid primarily because the participant had not answered all questions. The characteristics of respondents are presented in the tables 4.1, 4.2, 4.3. The maximum questionnaires received were from north zone (38.8%) followed by from west zone, east zone and least from south zone. Most of the participants (45.6%) are from the age group of 21-30 years. Further 65.7% of our participants are post graduated.

Table 4.1: Distribution of sample across different Zones

Zone	Frequency	Percentage
North	120	38.8
West	81	26.2
South	50	16.2
East	58	18.8

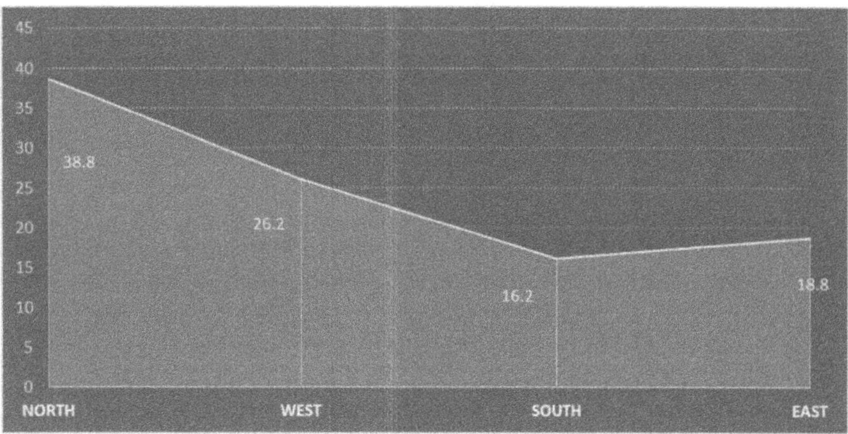

Figure 4.1: Distribution of sample across different zones.

Table 4.2: Distribution of sample across the different Age groups

Age group	Frequency	Percentage
21-30 years	141	45.6
31-40 years	123	39.8
41-50 years	32	10.4
51 years and above	13	4.2

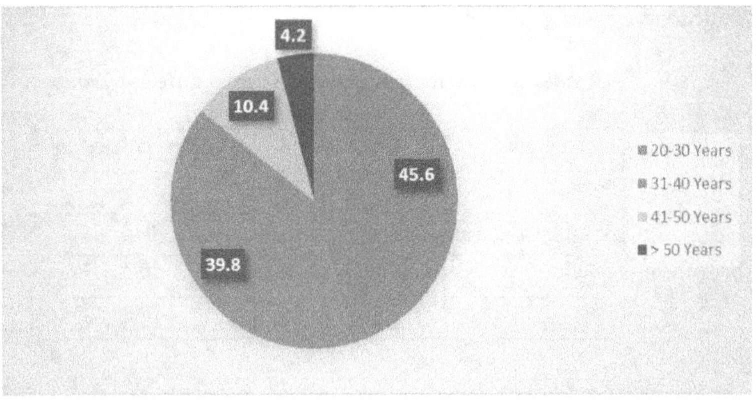

Figure 4.2: Distribution of sample across the different age groups

Table 4.3: Qualification of the Physiotherapists

Qualification	Frequency	Percentage
Diploma	10	3.2
Bachelor of Physiotherapy- 3 ½ years	5	1.6
Bachelor of Physiotherapy- 4 ½ years	91	29.4
Master of Physiotherapy	191	61.8
PhD	12	3.9

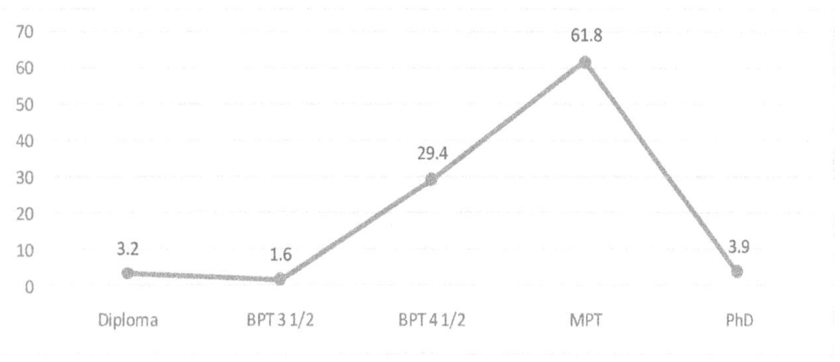

Figure 4.3: Qualification of Physiotherapists

The results show that around 57.9 % of the physiotherapists from our sample worked in in-patient as well as outpatient care setups. Furthermore, out of the total sample most of the physiotherapists were working as senior therapists (40.5%) followed by junior physiotherapists (28.5%). Almost 53.10% of the physiotherapists spent more than 50% of their job hours on patient care and up to 17.80% on administrative work. 68.10% of the therapists treat 6 or more patients/ day.

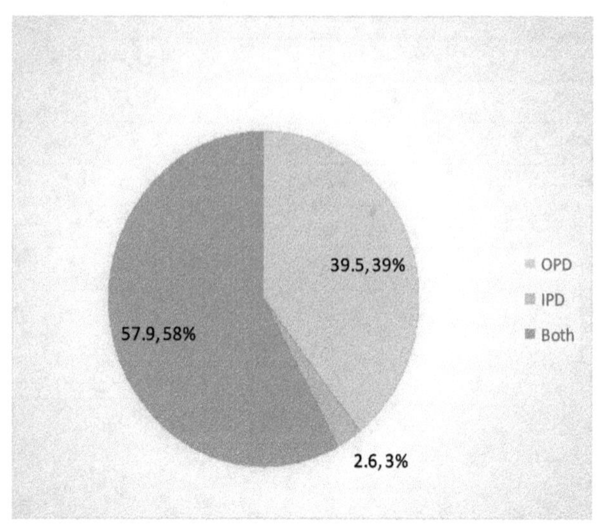

Figure 4.4: Working Set up

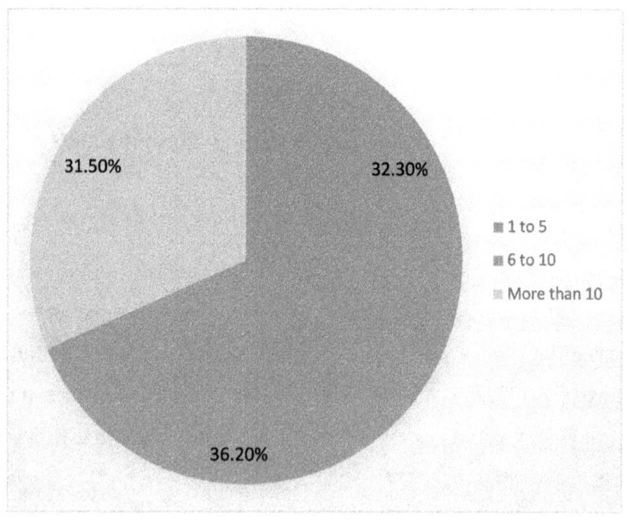

Figure 4.5: Number of patients treated/day

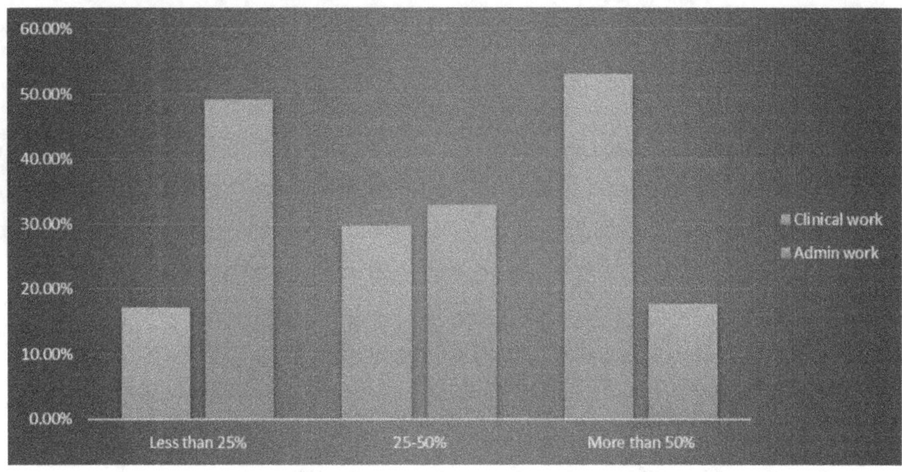

Figure 4.6: Time distribution of type of work

About 73.8% of the clinicians predominantly treated patients with musculoskeletal problems and 70.2% of the therapists used a combination of manual therapy and electrotherapy to treat their patients and almost 78% of the therapists followed LBP guidelines.

In this reliability study of the ABS - mp, Indian physiotherapists across a wide spectrum of demographics and from all four zones of the country participated. There was a 58 % return rate with the largest group from the north zone followed by the west zone. 80% of physiotherapists that responded were in the 21 - 40 year age-group and 70% of the physiotherapists had achieved higher education i.e. Masters or PhD degrees in the field of Physiotherapy. Additionally, our sample worked in different work settings, with 55% working in both Inpatient and Outpatient setups. 63.7% of the responding therapists treated six (6) or more patients which had mostly with musculoskeletal problems. Furthermore, they used a combination of electrotherapy and manual therapy to treat their patients. It was also observed that most of our sample followed international guidelines in their treatment approach to LBP.

As far as we know, this study is one of the first that has established the internal consistency of the ABS-mp questionnaire in physiotherapists working in different clinical set-ups across India. The ABS-mp Questionnaire is used worldwide to evaluate the attitude and beliefs towards the management in clinicians managing low back pain. Moreover, establishing reliability is an important first step in the evaluation of the validity of a measurement tool/questionnaire. More importantly, internal consistency establishes the agreement of items measuring the same construct, and it also determines if different subjects will respond in a consistent manner to similar questions posed by different clinicians. In this study, we found good internal consistency with a cronbach's alpha of 0.746 for the total ABS – mp score and 0.754 for the personal interaction and 0.76 for the treatment orientation sub-dimensions. In developing this questionnaire Pincus et al. (2006) using factor analysis found that overall the 19 items of the ABS-mp accounted for 56.4 % of the variance when administered to a sample of clinicians in the United Kingdom, suggesting good validity and reliability. Similarly, the results of this study suggest that in measuring attitudes and beliefs of Indian physiotherapists managing low back pain patients the ABS-mp can be used reliably.

The Attitude for Back pain scale for musculoskeletal practitioner (ABS-mp) is a valid measurement tool with good internal consistency when administered to a sample of diverse Indian Physiotherapist who treat and manage LBP. Hence this scale can be used reliably for future cross sectional studies in Indian Physiotherapists. (Refer Appendix IV for full article).

Reliability:

As stated earlier, we found good Internal Consistency of the questionnaire as Cronbach alpha of total ABS- mp was 0.746 and its sub- dimensions, Personal Interaction and Treatment orientated were 0.754 and 0.749 respectively. Thus, there was good agreement of items measuring the same construct, and furthermore a diverse sample subjects will respond in a consistent manner, thus ensuring stability of responses across items.

Table 4.4: Cronbach alpha of ABS- mp and its sub- dimensions; personal interaction and Treatment orientation.

Dimensions		Mean	Min.	Max	Range	Variance	Cronbach's Alpha	Cronbach's alpha based on Stand. Items
Total ABS-mp (N=19)	Item Mean	4.980	3.192	6.367	3.175	1.064	.746	.790
	Item Variances	2.243	1.192	3.388	2.196	.513		
Personal interaction (N= 13)	Item Mean	4.763	2.742	6.367	3.625	1.231	.754	.786
	Item Variances	2.302	1.192	3.388	2.196	.650		
Treatment orientation (N=6)	Item Mean	5.235	3.192	6.258	3.067	1.185	.749	.760
	Item Variances	2.118	1.437	2.756	1.319	.267		

4.2 ATTITUDES AND BELIEFS OF INDIAN PHYSIOTHERAPISTS

The overall scores suggest that on average Indian physiotherapists score high on the musculoskeletal version of the attitudes and beliefs scale (ABS – mp) and its sub-components. As seen in Table 4.5 mean ABS - mp total score was 95.12 ± 12.12. The mean score of personal interaction and treatment orientation domain was 63.41 ±8.41 and 31.71 ±5.06 respectively.

Table 4.5: Mean (±SD) of total score and sub-dimensions; treatment orientation and personal interaction along with maximum score

Domain/ Subdomain	Maximum Score	Mean	SD	Minimum	Maximum
Personal Interaction	**91**	**63.41**	**8.41**	**13.00**	**79.00**
LS	28	20.84	3.65	4.00	28.00
PS	28	17.48	4.29	4.00	28.00
CHS	21	14.87	2.60	3.00	21.00
CC	14	10.21	2.05	2.00	14.00
Treatment Orientation	**42**	**31.71**	**5.06**	**6.00**	**42.00**
RA	21	17.56	3.00	3.00	21.00
BM	21	14.15	2.93	3.00	21.00
Total ABS – mp	**133**	**95.12**	**12.12**	**19.00**	**121.00**

LS= Limitation on session (Max score= support unlimited session) (min.4- Max. 28)

PS= Psychological approach (Max score= supports psychological approach) (Min. 4- max. 28)

CHS= Connection to health care system (Max score= feel connected) (min. 3- Max.21)

CC= Confidence & concern (Max Score= confident) (Min. 2- Max.14)

RA= Re-activation (Max score= supports re-activation) (min. 3- Max.21)

BM= Biomedical (Max score= supports biomedical approach) (min. 3- Max.21)

Personal Interaction: Min - Max score = 13 – 91

Treatment Orientation: Min - Max score = 6 - 42

Total Abs - mp: Min - Max score = 19 - 133

4.3 ATTITUDES AND BELIEFS ACROSS DIFFERENT GEOGRAPHICAL ZONES:

The total ABS-mp score along with two domains, Treatment orientation and Personal Interaction was calculated to evaluate the attitude and beliefs across different geographical zones. The mean rank of each section is presented in Table 4.6.

Table 4.6: Mean rank and Kruskal Wallis (χ^2) test of total ABS-mp score and the sub-dimensions, personal interaction and treatment orientation across geographical zones.

Zones	Total Score			Treatment Orientation			Personal Interaction		
	Mean Rank	χ^2	p*	Mean Rank	χ^2	p*	Mean Rank	χ^2	p*
North (N= 120)	147.66			150.02			146.72		
West (N=81)	166.06	2.30	.512	158.92	.96	.810	167.26	2.62	.454
South (N= 50)	159.14			162.89			155.50		
East (N=58)	151.16			153.14			154.94		

As seen in table 4.6 and figure 4.7, there were no significant difference in the attitudes and beliefs of Physiotherapists with regards to the management of musculoskeletal conditions across the four zones.

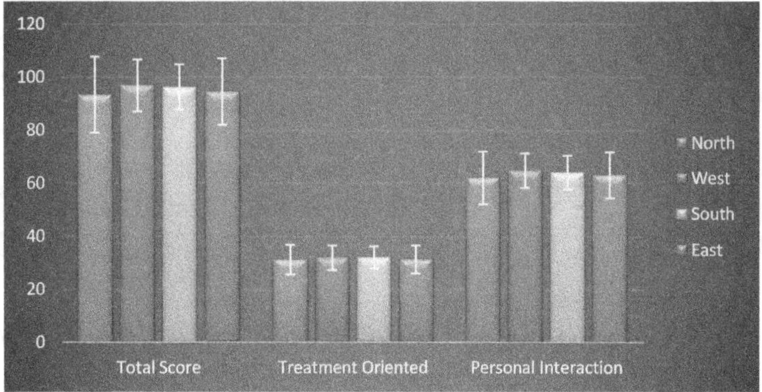

p>0.05

Figure 4.7: Mean (± SD) score total ABS-mp, attitude and belief score and its sub-dimensions, Personal interaction and Treatment orientation across different geographical zones.

4.4 ATTITUDES AND BELIEFS ACROSS GENDER:

The total ABS- mp score along with two domains Treatment orientation and Personal Interaction was calculated to evaluate the attitude and beliefs across gender. The mean rank of each section is presented in Table 4.7

Table 4.7: Mean rank and Mann Whitney 'U' test of total ABS-mp score and the sub-dimensions, personal interaction and treatment orientation across gender

Domain	Gender	N	Mean Rank	U value	p*
Total Score	Male	139	139.42	9649	.006
	Female	170	167.74		
Treatment Orientation	Male	139	143.65	1.02	.043
	Female	170	164.28		
Personal Interaction	Male	139	141.67	9.96	.018
	Female	170	165.90		

As seen in Table 4.7 and Figure 4.8, there was a significant difference in attitude and belief of Physiotherapists across gender. The female physiotherapists scored significantly more on the total better mean across all scores compared to male therapists with p < 0.05.

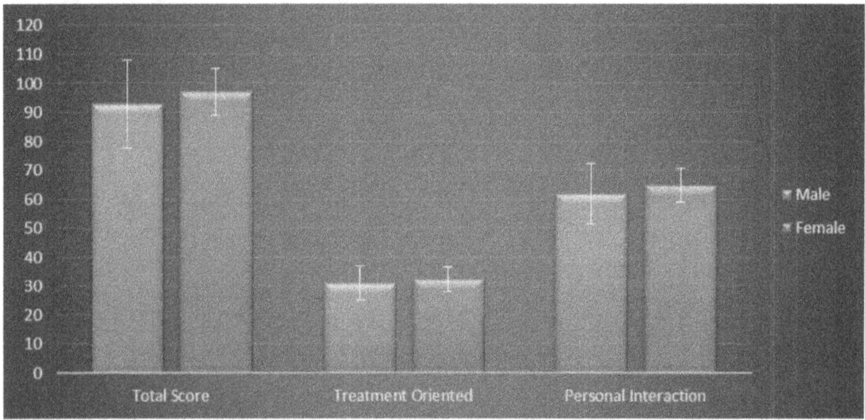

Figure 4.8: Mean (± SD) score total ABS-mp, attitude and belief score and its sub-dimensions, Personal interaction and Treatment orientation across gender.

4.5 ATTITUDES AND BELIEFS ACROSS EDUCATIONAL QUALIFICATIONS:

The total ABS-mp score along with two domains; Treatment orientation and Personal Interaction was calculated to evaluate the attitude and beliefs across educational qualifications. As the groups were small, they were collapsed under two groups of educational qualification of therapists i.e. under-graduate and post- graduate. The mean rank of each section is presented in Table 4.8.

Table 4.8: Mean rank and Mann Whitney 'U' test of total ABS-mp score and the sub-dimensions, treatment orientation and personal interaction across educational qualifications.

Qualification	Total Score			Treatment Orientation			Personal Interaction		
	Mean Rank	U value	p*	Mean Rank	U value	p	Mean Rank	U Value	p*
UG (106)	166.46			161.79			165.34		
PG (203)	142.22	8164	.023	144.43	8.61	.104	142.75	8.27	.035

As seen in Table 4.8 and Figure 4. 9, there was a significant difference in attitude and belief of Physiotherapists across educational qualification in total score and personal Interaction sub- domain but no significant difference in treatment orientation sub-domain. It showed that under graduate physiotherapists had significantly better attitude and belief than post graduate physiotherapists.

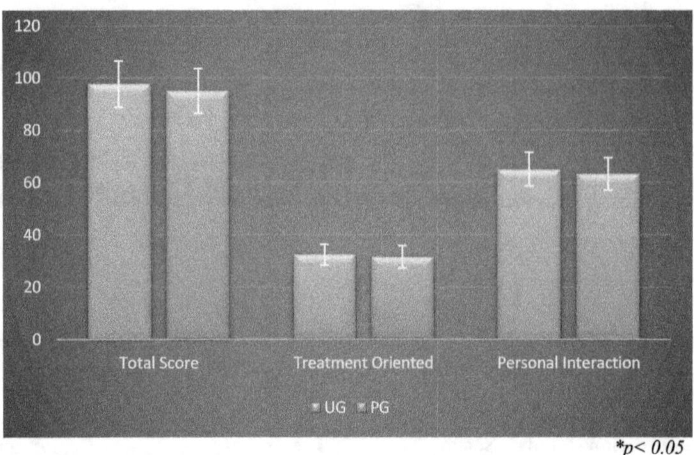

Figure 4.9: Mean (± SD) score total ABS-mp, attitude and belief score and its sub-dimensions, Personal interaction and Treatment orientation across qualification.

4.6 ATTITUDES AND BELIEFS ACROSS THERAPIST SPECIALIZATION:

The total ABS-mp score along with two domains; Treatment orientation and Personal Interaction was calculated to evaluate the attitude and beliefs across specialization of physiotherapists. The mean rank of each section is presented in Table 4.9.

Table 4.9: Mean rank and Kruskal wallis χ^2 test of total score ABS-mp and the sub-dimensions, treatment orientation and personal interaction across therapist specialization.

Specialization of therapist	Total Score			Treatment Orientation			Personal Interaction		
	Mean Rank	χ^2	p*	Mean Rank	χ^2	p*	Mean Rank	χ^2	p*
Musculoskeletal (N=179)	154.59			155.57			154.38		
Neurology (N= 52)	165.20	2.53	.283	159.39	1.44	.483	163.70	1.65	.439
Other (N=78)	131.44			134.98			136.46		

As Seen in Table 4.9 and Figure 4.10, there was no significant difference in attitude and beliefs of physiotherapists across the specializations. Further, the mean score of therapists with musculoskeletal, neurology and other specialization showed almost equal mean scores in both the domains.

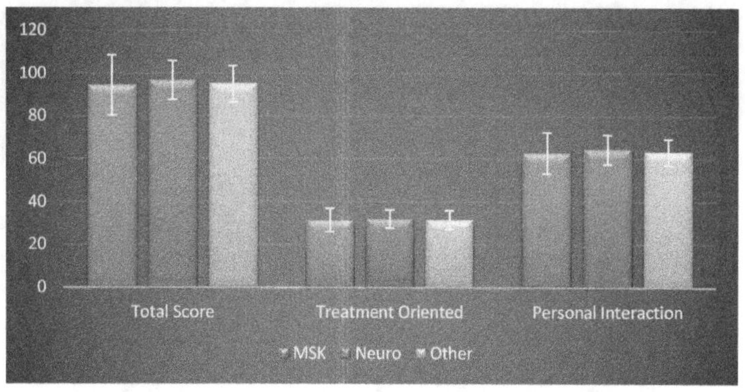

p> 0.05

Figure 4.10: Mean (± SD) score total ABS-mp, attitude and belief score and its sub-dimensions, Personal interaction and Treatment orientation across specialization.

4.7 ATTITUDES AND BELIEFS ACROSS TYPE OF INTERVENTIONS:

The total ABS-mp score along with two domains was calculated to evaluate the attitude and beliefs across therapists using different type of interventions. As the groups were small, they were collapsed under two groups' i.e manual therapy and both (combined). The mean rank of each section is presented in Table 4.10.

Table 4.10: Mean rank and Mann Whitney 'U' test of total score ABS-mp and the sub-dimensions, treatment orientation and personal interaction across type of interventions.

Interventions used	Total Score			Treatment Orientation			Personal Interaction		
	Mean Rank	U value	p*	Mean Rank	U value	p*	Mean Rank	U value	p*
Manual-Therapy (N= 63)	152.25			135.90			158.52		
		6473	.213		6.54	.628		6.07	.072
Combined (246)	141.03			145.65			139.26		

As seen in Table 4.10 and Figure 4.11, there was no significant difference in attitude and beliefs of physiotherapists using different types of treatment options.

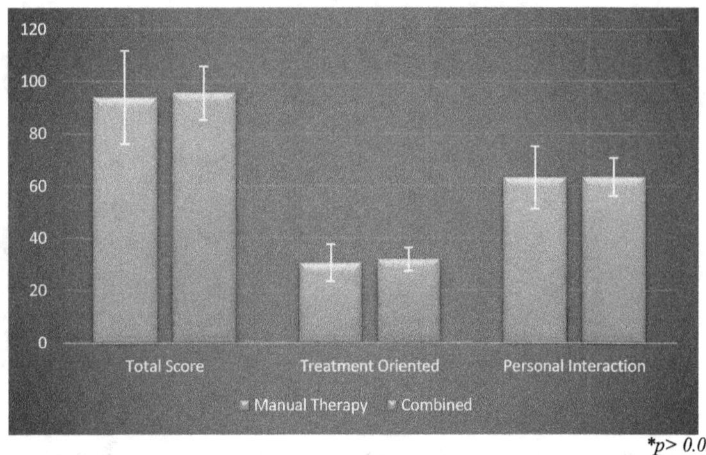

*p> 0.05

Figure 4.11: Mean (± SD) score total ABS-mp, attitude and belief score and its sub-dimensions, Personal interaction and Treatment orientation across interventions

4.8 ATTITUDES AND BELIEFS ACROSS PATIENT CARE SETUPS:

The total ABS-mp score along with two domains was calculated to evaluate the attitude and beliefs across therapists working in different type of patient care setups. As the IPD group was small, it was collapsed under both (OPD + IPD). The mean rank of each section is presented in Table 4.11.

Table 4.11: Mean rank and Mann Whitney 'U' test of total score ABS- mp and the sub-dimensions, treatment orientation and personal interaction across patient care setups.

Work setups	Total Score			Treatment Orientation			Personal Interaction		
	Mean Rank	U value	p*	Mean Rank	U value	p*	Mean Rank	U value	p*
OPD (N= 122)	158.05		.627	153.80		.848	156.86		.767
IPD+ Both (N= 187)	153.01	1.10		155.78	1.12		153.78	1.11	

(p> 0.05)

Table 4.11 and Figure 4.12 showed that there was no significant difference in attitude and beliefs of physiotherapists working in different patient care setups.

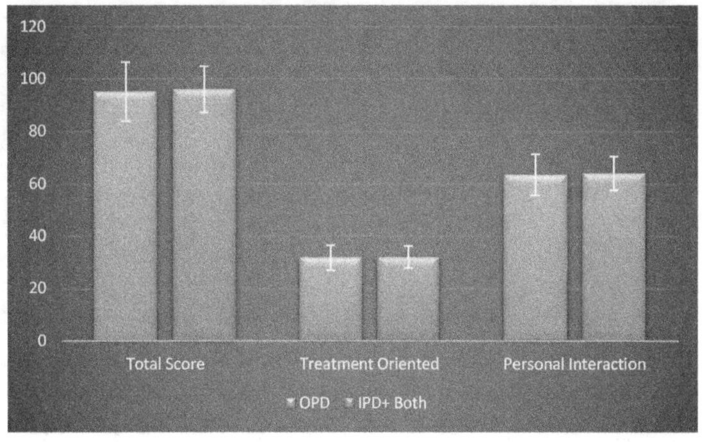

*p> 0.05

Figure 4.12: Mean (±SD) score total ABS-mp, attitude and belief score and its sub-dimensions, Personal interaction and Treatment orientation across work set up

4.9 ATTITUDES AND BELIEFS ACROSS USE OF GUIDELINE:

The total ABS-mp score of two domains was calculated to evaluate the attitude and beliefs across therapists following and not following international guidelines. The mean rank of each section is presented in Table 4.12.

Table 4.12: Mean rank and Mann- Whitney 'U' test of total score ABS- mp and the sub-dimensions, treatment orientation and personal interaction across use of guidelines.

Domain	follow Guidelines	N	Mean Rank	U- value	p*
Total Score	Yes	242	156.52		
	No	67	147.62	7848.5	.462
Treatment Orientation	Yes	242	155.83		
	No	67	149.96	8.012	.627
Personal interaction	Yes	242	155.62		
	No	67	150.69	8.064	.684

As seen in Table 4.12 and Figure 4.13, there was no significant difference in attitude and beliefs of physiotherapists following and not following the international guidelines.

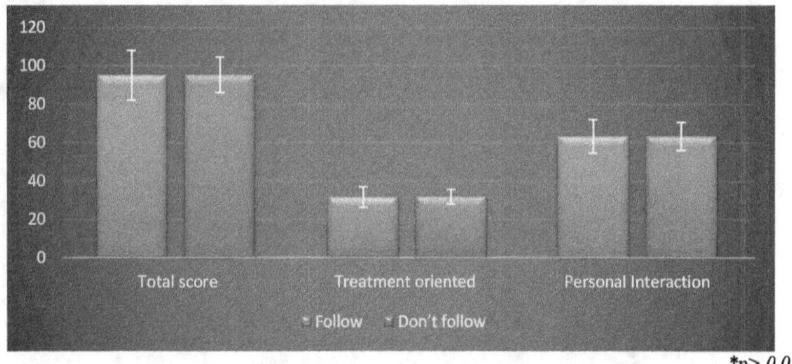

*p> 0.05

Figure 4.13: Mean (±SD) score total ABS-mp, attitude and belief score and its sub-dimensions, Personal interaction and Treatment orientation across use of guidelines

CHAPTER FIVE: DISCUSSION

Low Back Pain (LBP) and related disability remain a prevalent and great economic burden on patients (Burton et al. 2006). Clearly, the management of LBP is first and foremost dependent on the clinical skills of a physiotherapist, however it is largely also dependent on the attitude and belief of the clinicians. This study, to the best of our knowledge, is the only study that has addressed factors associated with the attitudes and beliefs of Indian physiotherapist's with regards to the management of LBP. The primary aim of this study was to gather information from Indian Physiotherapists regarding the attitudinal factors that guide the management of LBP, and secondly and more importantly their use of psychological and/or biomedical approaches, connection to the health care system, use of guidelines, assessments, treatment recommendations, number of treatments, etc. Data from this study provides significant insights into the mode of practice of Indian Physiotherapist with regards to the course and type of approach, longevity of treatment and their views on when patients should return to work etc.

Indian Physiotherapists from all four zones of India with a wide spectrum of demographics, and who were representative of physiotherapy profession, participated in this cross sectional study. The largest number of participants was from north zone, with 38.8 % followed by west zone. 80% of Physiotherapists that responded were in the 21 - 40 year age group and 65.7% of the physiotherapists had achieved higher education i.e. Masters and/or PhD degree in the field of Physiotherapy. Additionally, therapists worked in different work settings, with 55% working in both Inpatient and Outpatient setups and 63.7% of the responding therapists treated six (6) or more patients that had primarily musculoskeletal problems. Furthermore, most of them (59.9%) used a combination of electrotherapy and manual therapy to treat their patients, and followed international guidelines in their treatment approach to LBP.

Overall, it was observed that Indian physiotherapists scored moderately high on the ABS-mp scale, including its sub-domains. This suggests that Indian physiotherapists rely to a great extent on their willingness to engage patients in the management of their LBP. This inclusion extended to their willingness to address the psychological problems suffered by their patients, the limitation of number of treatments, referrals to other specialities/experts, the use of the biomedical approach and their views and focus on the patients return to activity. The result suggests that Indian physios support more sessions, believe in using a psychological approach to some extent, are fairly confident about their clinical competence and have some knowledge of the healthcare system. Similar findings have been reported in a systematic review of quantitative and qualitative studies. It is reported that clinicians that followed a strong biomedical approach in their treatment of LBP advised patients to limit their activities and delayed their return to work (Gardner T, Refshauge K, Smith L, McAuley J, Hubscher M, Godall S (2017).

Physiotherapists across geographical zones had similar attitudes and beliefs with regards to managing LBP patients. This was an interesting finding given the diversity of India with regards to professional education. However, a review of the syllabus taught across physiotherapy institutions revealed that the theoretical and clinical components were fairly similar, and more importantly the health care delivery systems were the same across the country (refer to Appendix V - Rajiv Gandhi University of Health Sciences Bangalore, University of Delhi, Maharashtra University of Health Sciences, West Bengal University of health sciences). Accordingly, it is not surprising that no significant differences were found in therapists that worked in different organizational setups, or had different specializations, used guidelines or not, or the type of interventions used essentially, therapists were exposed to similar academic experiences and they all followed similar international guidelines. (WCPT 2016)

It is surprising that there was no significant difference in attitudes and beliefs across patient care setups. It is possible that these non – significant differences were because most of our sample worked in both OPD and IPD settings. Thus, they are exposed to more equitable and open environment where other health care professionals work alongside to manage the patient. This definitely influences the attitude and belief of the therapists in positive way. Further, patient discharged from the in-patient department is usually advised to continue physiotherapy at the same hospital / organization.

The results also revealed significant differences in attitudes and beliefs by gender and the physiotherapist's qualifications. It was observed that males scored lesser than females across all attitude dimensions, suggesting that female therapists were more likely to use a psychological approach, recommend more treatment sessions. Similarly, attitude and belief of the therapists across educational qualification had significant difference. Physiotherapists with undergraduate degrees were significantly better than therapists with regards to their attitude and beliefs in managing patients with low back pain. This suggests that younger therapists were more willing to listen to their patients, while therapists with postgraduate degrees assumed that they were more knowledgeable and thus, were less likely to consider the opinion of their patients.

As the results showed better attitude and belief in female physiotherapists and in entry level professionals, we here by accept our alternate hypotheses regarding difference in attitude and belief across gender and educational qualification. However, there was no significant difference in attitude and belief across various zones, specialisation and adherence to guideline or not. Therefore, we hereby accept our null hypothesis regarding no difference in attitude and belief across these domains.

It is important to keep in mind that there are several limitations of this study. The first and foremost is the limited sample size. Thus, generalizability of the results and inferences thereof, should be interpreted and embellished with caution. In addition, our study sample was geographically skewed as it had more subjects from the north zone. Future studies should make an attempt to recruit more participant from other zones using stratified sampling. Additionally, studies in the future should address the influence/impact of cultural factors and/or geographical specific attitudes and beliefs, which possibly have a significant impact on clinical decision making in the management of a number of health conditions.

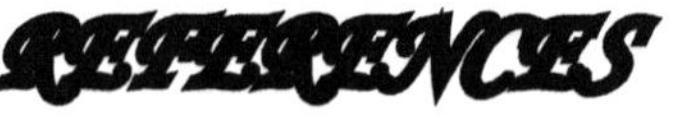

REFERENCES

1. Andersson G.B. Epidemiological features of chronic low-back pain. Lancet 1999; 354: 581-585.

2. "Low Back Pain Fact Sheet". National Institute of Neurological Disorders and stroke https://www.ninds.nih.gov/Disorders/Patients

3. Australian Acute Musculoskeletal Pain Guidelines Group. Evidence based management of acute pain. Acute low back pain. 2003.

4. Balagué, F., Mannion, A.F., Pellisé, F. and Cedraschi, C. Non-Specific Low Back Pain. Lancet. 2012; 19: 379

5. Bishop A, Foster NE. Do physical therapists in the United Kingdom recognize psychosocial factors in patients with acute low back pain? Spine. 2005; 30: 1316–22.

6. Buchbinder R, Jolley D. Effects of a media campaign on back beliefs is sustained 3 years after its cessation. Spine (Phila Pa 1976). 2005; 30(11):1323-30.

7. Casazza, BA (15 February 2012). "Diagnosis and treatment of acute low back pain". *American Family Physician*. 85 (4): 343–50

8. Chou, R., Qaseem, A., et al.. (2007) Diagnosis and Treatment of Low Back Pain: A Joint Clinical Practice Guideline from the American College of Physicians and the American Pain Society. Annals of Internal Medicine, 147, 478-491.

9. Daykin AR, Richardson B. Physiotherapists' pain beliefs and their influence on the management of patients with chronic low back pain. Spine. 2004; 29:783–95.

10. Fidvi, N. and May, S. Physiotherapy management of low back pain in India — a survey of self-reported practice. Physiother. Res. Int 2010, 15: 150–159.

11. Foster NE, Pincus T, Underwood MR, et al. Understanding the process of care for musculoskeletal conditions: why a biomedical approach is inadequate. Rheumatism. 2003; 42: 401–440.

12.	Gardner T, Refshauge K, Smith L, McAuley J, Hübscher M, Goodall S. Physiotherapists' beliefs and attitudes influence clinical practice in chronic low back pain: a systematic review of quantitative and qualitative studies. J Physiother. 2017; 63(3):132-143.

13.	Goubert L, Crombez G, Hermans D, Vanderstraeten G, et al.. Implicit attitude towards pictures of back-stressing activities in painfree subjects and patients with low back pain: an effective priming study. Eur J Pain. 2003;7:33–47.

14.	Harvey E, Burton AK, Klaber-Moffett J, Breen AC. Spinal manipulation for low-back pain: a treatment package agreed by the UK chiropractic, osteopathy and physiotherapy professional associations. Manual Therapy 2003;8:46–51.

15.	Hay EM, Mullis R, Lewis M, Vohora K, Main CJ, Watson P, et al.. Comparison of physical treatments versus a brief pain-management programme for back pain in primary care: a randomised clinical trial in physiotherapy practice. Lancet 2005;365:2024–30.

16.	Houben RM, Vlaeyen JW, Peters M, Ostelo RW, Wolters PM, Stomp-van den Berg SG. Health care providers' attitudes and beliefs towards common low back pain: factor structure and psychometric properties of the HC-PAIRS. Clin J Pain. 2004;20(1):37-44.

17.	Houben RMA, Gijsen A, Peterson J, deJong PJ, Vlaeyen JWS. Do health care providers' attitudes towards back pain predict their treatment recommendations? Differential predictive validity of implicit and explicit attitude measures. Pain 2005b; 114:491–8.

18.	Houben RMA, Vlaeyen JWS, Peters M, Ostelo RWJG, Wolters PMJC, Stomp-van den Berg SGM. Health care provider's attitudes and beliefs towards common low back pain: factor structure and psychometric properties of the HC-PAIRS. Clinical Journal of Pain 2004; 20:37–44.

19.	Innes, S.I., Werth, P.D., Tuchin, P.J. *et al.* Attitudes and beliefs of Australian chiropractors' about managing back pain: a cross-sectional study. *Chiropr Man Therap 2015,* **23,** 17

20.	Jensen, MP. and Karoly, P. Notes on the Survey of Pain Attitudes (SOPA): original (24-item) and revised (35-item) versions (unpublished manuscript), Arizona State University, Tempe. AZ, 1987.

21.	Liddle SD, Baxter GD, Gracey JH. Chronic low back pain: patients' experiences, opinions and expectations for clinical management. Disabil Rehabil. 2007; 29(24):1899–1909.

22.	Linton SJ, Vlaeyen J, Ostelo R. The back pain beliefs of health care providers: are we fear-avoidant? J Occup Rehabil. 2002; 12: 223–32.

23.	Maniadakis N, Gray A. The economic burden of back pain in the UK. Pain 2000; 84:95–103.

24.	 Melloh M, Röder C, Elfering A, Theis JC, Müller U, Staub LP, et al.. Differences across health care systems in outcome and cost-utility of surgical and conservative treatment of chronic low back pain: a study protocol. BMC Musculoskelet Disord. 2008; 9:81.

25.	Meucci, Rodrigo Dalke, Anaclaudia Gastal Fassa, and Neice Muller Xavier Faria. Prevalence of chronic low back pain: systematic review. Revista de saude publica. 2015: 49

26.	Norelee Kennedy, John Healy, and Kieran O'Sullivan The beliefs of third-level healthcare students towards low-back pain. Pain Research and Treatment. 2014; Article ID 675915.

27.	Ostelo RW, Stomp-van den Berg SG, Vlaeyen JW, Wolters PM, de Vet HC. Health care provider's attitudes and beliefs towards chronic low back pain: the development of a questionnaire. Man Ther. 2003; 8: 214–22.

28.	Philadelphia Panel. Philadelphia Panel evidence-based clinical practice guidelines on selected rehabilitation interventions for low back pain. Phys Ther. 2001;81(10):1641-74.

29.	Pincus T, Kent P, Bronfort G, Loisel P, Pransky G, Hartvigsen J. 25 Years with the Biopsychosocial model of Low Back Pain – Is it time to celebrate? Spine. 2013; 38(24):2118–23.

30.   Pincus T, Vogel S, Burton AK, Santos R, Field AP. Fear avoidance and prognosis in low back pain: a systematic review and synthesis of current evidence. Arthritis Rheum. 2006;54(12):3999-4010.

31.   Pincus T, Vogel S, Santos R, Breen A, Foster NE, Underwood MR. The Attitudes to Back Pain Scale in musculoskeletal practitioners (ABS-mp); The development and testing of a new questionnaire. Clin J Pain. 2006; 22: 378–86.

32.   Rainville J, Bagnall D, Phalen L. Health care providers' attitudes and beliefs about functional impairments and chronic back pain. Clinical Journal of Pain 1995; 11:287–95.

33.   Rainville J, Carlson N, Polatin P, et al.. Exploration of physicians' recommendations for activities in chronic low back pain. Spine. 2000; 25: 2210–2220.

34.   Riley, J.F., Ahern. D.K. and Follick, M.J., Chronic pain and lunctionalimpairment: assessing beliefs about their relationship. Arch.Phys. Med. Rehabil. 1988; 69: 579-582.

35.   Savigny P, Kuntze S, Watson P, Underwood M, Ritchie G, Cotterell M, Hill D, Browne N, Buchanan E, Coffey P, Dixon P, Drummond C, Flanagan M, Greenough C, Griffiths M, Halliday-Bell J, Hettinga D, Vogel S, Walsh D. Low Back Pain: early management of persistent non-specific low back pain. London: National Collaborating Centre for Primary Care and Royal College of General Practitioners; 2009.

36.   Schwartz. D.P. DeGood, D.E. and Shutty. M.S. Direct assessment of beliefs and attitudes of chronic pain patients. Arch. Phys. Med.Rehahil. 1985; 66: 806-809.

37.   Shutty. MS., DeGood. D.E. and Tuttle. D.H., Chronic pain patients'beliefs about their pain and treatment outcomes. Arch. Phys.Med. Rehahil. 1990; 76: 128-332.

38.   Strong J, Ashton R, Chant D. The Measurement of attitudes towards and beliefs about pain. PAIN. 1992; 48: 227-236.

39.   Strong, J., Ashton, R. Cramond. T. and Chant, D. Pain intensity, attitudes and function in back pain patients. Aust. Occup. Ther.J. 1990; 37: 179-183.

40.   Supreet Bindra, Sinha A.G.K & Benjamin A.I. Epidemiology of Low Back Pain in Indian Population: A Review; International Journal of Basic and Applied Medical Sciences. 2015; 5 (1): 166-179

41.   Tamar Pincusa, Nadine E Foster, Steven Vogel, Rita Santos, Alan Breend, & Martin Underwood. Attitudes to back pain amongst musculoskeletal practitioners: A comparison of professional groups and practice settings using the ABS-mp. Manual Therapy. 2007; 12: 167–175.

42.   Vlaeyen JW, Linton SJ. Are we 'fear-avoidant'? Pain. 2006; 124:240–1.

43.   Walker BF. The prevalence of low back pain: systematic review of the literature from 1966 to 1998, Clinical Spine Surgery, 2000

44.   Williams. D.A. and Thorn, B.E., An empirical assessment of pain beliefs. Pain. 1989; 36: 351-358.

CHAPTER SIX: CONCLUSION

A clinician's attitudes and beliefs are an integral part in the management of patients with LBP, and to the best of our knowledge, this is the only study that has examined these factors in Indian Physiotherapists. Clinical decision making is an interactive process, and ideally takes into consideration, both the clinician's and the patient's attitudes and beliefs. For an example, a clinician's belief regarding treatment orientation and fear avoidance to movement will influence the physiotherapist to use more passive forms of treatment and advice patients to refrain from activity and delay their return to work. This approach, interestingly will influence the patient's attitudes, beliefs, and expectations with regards to the cause of their low back pain and reinforce how it should be managed, and consequently impact upon the physiotherapist's treatment plan – setting up a vicious cycle (Gardner et al., 2017; Houben et al., 2005; Bishop et al., 2006)).

It is noteworthy that Indian physiotherapist involved in the management of LBP demonstrate, at minimum, demonstrated a willingness to engage with the patient's affective state, to increase the number of therapy sessions, refer patients to other experts if they do not get better, and they demonstrated an increased confidence in their clinical competency. However, a small percentage of clinicians who primarily used a bio-medical approach, advised their patients to delay their return to work etc. Interestingly, this trend was observed more in female therapists and physiotherapists who had entry level degrees instead of postgraduate degrees.

Inferences from the results of the current study can be used as baseline data for making several new policies and procedures related to the management of this very prevalent and disabling musculoskeletal condition, especially given the biological and cultural diversity of our patient population. The importance of attitudes and beliefs in the management of LBP, as highlighted in this study, will help create standardised, baseline treatment guidelines. This endeavour is particularly of importance given the significant move of the global, as well as the Indian health systems towards evidence-informed practice. The uniformity and standardization of LBP treatment will help clinicians rehabilitate their patients comprehensively and effectively, in a relatively shorter period of time. This would consequently reduce lost time due to disability and by extension reduce the economic burden – both to the patient as well as to society.

Finally, the results of the current study has given a new and significant insights with regards to the attitudes and beliefs of Indian physiotherapists managing LBP. In addition to its contribution to current literature in this domain, the information gleamed from this study will be beneficial to several stakeholders, including policy makers and other health care professionals involved in the management of LBP. Importantly, policy makers will be able to utilize this knowledge to create new, uniform nationwide policies to manage LBP efficiently across patient treatment setups, specialisations and geographical boundaries.